Guidelines
for
Cholera
Control

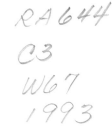

World Health Organization
Geneva
1993

WHO Library Cataloguing in Publication Data
Guidelines for cholera control.

1. Cholera — prevention & control — handbooks

ISBN 92 4 154449 X   (NLM Classification: WC 39)

PRINTED IN SWITZERLAND

92/9366 - Strategic - 7500

Contents

Preface

These guidelines have been prepared by the Global Task Force on Cholera Control of the World Health Organization to help managers of national diarrhoeal disease control programmes and others responsible for implementing cholera control activities. They may also be useful to international, bilateral, and non-governmental agencies in deciding on appropriate means of assisting countries to control cholera outbreaks.

The WHO Global Task Force on Cholera Control was created in April 1991, and is comprised of representatives from the Programme for Control of Diarrhoeal Diseases, the Community Water Supply and Sanitation unit, the Food Safety programme, the Strengthening of Epidemiological and Statistical Services unit, the Office of Information, the Microbiology and Immunology Support Services unit, the Office of External Coordination, the Division of Health Education, the Division of Emergency Relief Operations, and the Action Programme on Essential Drugs. A staff member of the United Nations Children's Fund (UNICEF) regularly contributes to the work of the Task Force.

Additional information may be obtained by contacting the Programme for Control of Diarrhoeal Diseases, World Health Organization, 1211 Geneva 27, Switzerland.

Acknowledgements

The important contributions of WHO's Community Water Supply and Sanitation unit to this publication are gratefully acknowledged, as are those of the other members of the Global Task Force on Cholera Control and the Geneva office of the United Nations Children's Fund (UNICEF).

The laboratory methods described in Annex 5 are based on the *Manual for laboratory investigations of acute enteric infections.*[1] Dr John Albert of the International Centre for Diarrhoeal Disease Research, Bangladesh, Dr Dhiman Barua formerly of the Programme for Control of Diarrhoeal Diseases, World Health Organization, Geneva, Switzerland, Dr Bradford Kay of Johns Hopkins University School of Hygiene and Public Health, Baltimore, MD, USA, and Dr Kaye Wachsmuth of the Centers for Disease Control, Atlanta, GA, USA assisted in preparing the guidelines.

WHO also appreciates the contributions of Dr Paul A. Blake, Dr Mitchell Cohen, Dr Roger I. Glass, Dr Allen Ries, Dr Robert Tauxe, Dr Duc Vugia, and Dr Todd Weber of the Centers for Disease Control, Atlanta, GA, USA, Dr Bruce Dick of the International Federation of Red Cross and Red Crescent Societies, Geneva, Switzerland, Dr Ann Dawson and Dr Roger Skinner of the Department of Health, London, England, Dr Sandy Cairncross of the London School of Hygiene and Tropical Medicine, London, England, Dr Jamie Bartram of the Robens Institute, University of Surrey, Guildford, England, Professor John Pickford of Loughborough University of Technology, Loughborough, England, Dr John Kvenberg of the United States Food and Drug Administration, Washington, DC, USA, and Dr Eugene Rice of the United States Environmental Protection Administration, Washington, DC, USA, whose suggestions helped to make this a more practical publication.

---

[1] *Manual for laboratory investigations of acute enteric infections.* Geneva, World Health Organization, 1987 (unpublished WHO document CDD/83.3 Rev. 1, available on request from the Programme for Control of Diarrhoeal Diseases, World Health Organization, 1211 Geneva 27, Switzerland).

1
Introduction

Cholera has spread widely since 1961 and now affects at least 98 countries. Extensive experience has shown that the introduction of cholera into a country cannot be prevented; its spread *within* a country, however, *can* be contained by appropriate control measures.

During the past three decades, intensive research has contributed substantially to our understanding of the epidemiology and clinical management of cholera. It is now known that:

- in more than 90% of cases cholera is mild, and may therefore be difficult to distinguish from other types of acute diarrhoeal disease;
- asymptomatic carriers of the disease are common;
- improved treatment, in most cases by oral rehydration therapy, can reduce case fatality rates for cholera to less than 1%;
- where cholera is present but not epidemic, it causes fewer than 5% of all cases of acute diarrhoea;
- vaccination, mass chemoprophylaxis, and *cordon sanitaire* are ineffective in preventing or controlling outbreaks;
- care in drinking and eating habits, safe disposal of excreta, and personal cleanliness are the most effective ways for individuals to reduce the risk of cholera.

Because cholera can be an acute public health problem, with the potential to spread quickly and cause many deaths, special attention must be given to surveillance and control. These guidelines provide information to assist national diarrhoea control programmes, emergency task forces, and others in their efforts to control cholera.

2
About cholera

Most cholera infections are mild; patients may have no symptoms or only mild diarrhoea. In a minority of cases, however, there is rapid onset of severe watery diarrhoea and vomiting, resulting in the loss of large amounts of fluid and salts from the body. Patients become thirsty, stop urinating, and quickly become weak and dehydrated. Patients with severe cholera often complain of cramps in the stomach, arms, or legs.

All cases of cholera should be treated immediately. If treatment is delayed or inadequate, death from dehydration and circulatory collapse may follow very shortly.

There are more than 60 serogroups of *Vibrio cholerae*, but only serogroup O1 causes cholera. *Vibrio cholerae* O1 occurs as two biotypes — classical and El Tor. Each biotype also occurs as two serotypes — Ogawa and Inaba. The El Tor biotype has caused almost all of the recent cholera outbreaks, although cases caused by the classical biotype still occur on the Indian subcontinent. The El Tor biotype also causes a higher proportion of asymptomatic infections than the classical biotype and survives longer in the environment. It can live in association with certain aquatic plants and animals, making water an important reservoir for infection.

Cholera is acquired by the ingestion of an infectious dose of cholera vibrios. Faecally contaminated water is usually the vehicle for transmission of infection, either directly or through the contamination of food. Food may also be contaminated by the soiled hands of infected persons.

The dose of *Vibrio cholerae* O1 required to produce illness depends on the susceptibility of the individual. It can be affected by the level of acidity in the stomach (the vibrio is destroyed at pH 4.5 or lower), and by immunity produced by prior infection with *Vibrio cholerae* O1. In endemic areas, breast-feeding protects infants and young children.

Box 1. Common sources of infection

- **Drinking-water**

  that has been contaminated at its source (e.g. by faecally contaminated surface water entering an incompletely sealed well) or during storage (e.g. by contact with hands soiled by faeces), and ice made from contaminated water.

- **Food contaminated during or after preparation**

  e.g. milk, cooked rice, lentils, potatoes, beans, eggs, and chicken.

- **Seafood**

  particularly shellfish, taken from contaminated water and eaten raw or insufficiently cooked.

- **Fruit and vegetables**

  grown at or near ground level and fertilized with night-soil, irrigated with water containing human waste, or "freshened" with contaminated water, and then eaten raw.

3
Preventing cholera

The only sure means of protection against cholera epidemics are adequate water supplies and sanitation.

3.1 Ensuring a safe water supply

Access to safe water is a basic requirement for health, made more critical when cholera threatens. Since contaminated water is the usual source of cholera infection, all efforts must be made to provide safe drinking-water, as well as safe water for food preparation and bathing. The supply of water must be of good quality, affordable, and available to all — continuously and in sufficient quantity for all domestic purposes.

Box 2. Recommended chlorine levels in water distribution systems in areas affected by cholera

The minimum levels of free residual chlorine necessary for safe water are:

- at all sampling points in a piped water system .... 0.5 mg/litre

- at standposts in systems with standposts .... 1.0 mg/litre

- in tanker trucks, at filling .... 2.0 mg/litre

Active monitoring is required to ensure that these minimum levels of chlorine are maintained.

In urban areas, properly treated drinking-water should be made available to the entire population through a piped system, at standposts, or from tanker trucks. In rural areas, where there is no source of treated water and where water from tube wells, protected dug wells, or protected springs is not available, people must be taught that water can be made safe at home by bringing it to a vigorous, rolling boil or by adding a chlorine-releasing chemical.

A supply of suitable chemicals for treating water, and narrow-mouthed pots with covers for storing water, are helpful in reducing secondary transmission of cholera within a family. Household filtration of water can also help to eliminate the vibrio, but should always be followed by disinfection with chlorine or by boiling. (Further information on providing safe water in communities and individual homes can be found in *Fact sheets on environmental sanitation for cholera control*.[1])

Boiling is an effective method of water sterilization, but is not practical for the needs of most populations, especially when fuel is scarce. The method is expensive and should be recommended chiefly for emergency situations when the disinfection of water by chlorination or other methods is not possible.

Box 3. Making water safe by boiling

To make water safe for drinking and other uses, bring water to a vigorous, rolling boil and keep it boiling for 1 minute. This will kill, or inactivate, *Vibrio cholerae* O1 and most other organisms that cause diarrhoea.

Even when drinking-water is safe, infection may still be transmitted by contaminated surface water used for bathing or for washing cooking utensils. When surface water is contaminated, as confirmed by laboratory tests, appropriate measures — including closing affected areas — should be taken to reduce the danger of infection. Indeed, special care should be given to *any* source of water shown to be contaminated. The water should be made safe or, if this is not possible, an alternative water source should be provided.

---

[1] *Fact sheets on environmental sanitation for cholera control*. Geneva, Health World Organization (in preparation). Will be available on request from Community Water Supply and Sanitation, World Health Organization, 1211 Geneva 27, Switzerland.

Box 4. Making water safe by chlorination

The following guidelines should be translated into messages that take appropriate account of locally available products and measuring devices, and of whether the instructions are for home or institutional use.

Make a stock solution of chlorine (1% concentration by weight of available chlorine). Add to 1 litre of water:

Product *(percent concentration by weight of available chlorine)*	*Amount*
Calcium hypochlorite (70%)	15 g
or	
Bleaching powder or chlorinated lime (30%)	33 g
or	
Sodium hypochlorite (5%)	250 ml
or	
Sodium hypochlorite (10%)	110 ml

If products with these concentrations of chlorine are not available in the local market, adjust the amount used according to the available concentrations.

Store the stock solution in a cool place in a closed container that does not admit light. The stock solution loses effectiveness with time and must be used no later than one month after it has been made.

Use the stock solution to make safe water. Add water to the stock solution to ensure proper mixing:

Water	added to	*Stock solution*
1 litre		0.6 ml or 3 drops
10 litres		6 ml
100 litres		60 ml

Allow the chlorinated water to stand for at least 30 minutes before using it. The residual chlorine level after 30 minutes should be between 0.2 and 0.5 mg/litre.

If the water is turbid (not clear, with a lot of suspended solid matter):

- filter it before chlorination, or

- boil it vigorously (as indicated in Box 3) instead of treating it by chlorination.

3.2 Sanitation

Good sanitation can markedly reduce the risk of transmission of intestinal pathogens, including cholera vibrios; this is especially true where the lack of good sanitation may lead to contamination of clean water sources. High priority should be given to observing the basic principles of sanitary human waste disposal, as well as to ensuring the availability of safe water supplies.

Appropriate facilities for human waste disposal are a basic need of all communities; in the absence of such facilities there is a high risk of cholera. Sanitary systems that are appropriate for the local conditions should be constructed with the cooperation of the community. (Designs for latrine construction in different types of soils and climatic conditions can be found in the WHO publication, *A guide to the development of on-site sanitation.*[1] See also Annex 1 for instructions on building a ventilated improved pit latrine.)

People will need to be taught how to use latrines, about the dangers of defecating on the ground, or in or near water, and about the importance of thorough hand-washing with soap or ash after any contact with excreta. The disposal of children's excreta in latrines needs to be emphasized.

When large groups of people congregate, for fairs, funerals, religious festivals, etc., particular care must be taken to ensure the safe disposal of human waste and the provision of adequate facilities for hand-washing.

---

[1] Franceys R, Pickford J, Reed R. *A guide to the development of on-site sanitation.* Geneva, World Health Organization, 1992.

Box 5. Preparing an emergency pit latrine

In an emergency, while a more permanent latrine is being built, a simple pit can be dug as a *temporary* solution for the disposal of human excreta. It should measure 0.3 x 0.3 metre, have a depth of 0.5 metre, and be at least 30 metres from a well or other source of drinking-water. Where possible, the pit should be at least 6 metres from the nearest house. It should not be located uphill from the water source or dug in marshy soil. The bottom of the pit should never penetrate the groundwater table.

After each use, a layer of soil should be laid down in the pit. In an area affected by cholera, the pit should also be coated each day with a layer of unslaked lime.

3.3 Food safety

Since food can be an important vehicle for disease organisms, each country should establish adequate controls for the handling and processing of food through a national programme on food safety.

Health education activities, which should be intensified where there is a threat of cholera, should stress the importance of:

- avoiding raw food (exception: undamaged fruits and vegetables from which the peel can be removed are safe if hygienically handled);
- cooking food until it is hot throughout;
- eating food while it is still hot, or reheating it thoroughly before eating;
- washing and thoroughly drying all cooking and serving utensils after use;
- handling and preparing food in a way that reduces the risk of contamination (e.g. cooked food and eating utensils should be kept separate from uncooked foods and potentially contaminated utensils); and
- washing hands thoroughly with soap (or ash) after defecating, or after contact with faecal matter, and before preparing or eating food, or feeding children.

Box 6. WHO Centres for Environmental Health

For additional information and assistance on water supply and sanitation measures contact:

Regional Centre for Environmental Health Activities (CEHA)
P.O. Box 926967
Amman
Jordan

Centre for Promotion of Environment Planning and Applied
    Sciences (PEPAS)
P.O. Box 12550
Kuala Lumpur 50782
Malaysia

Centro Panamericano de Ingenieria Sanitaria y Ciencias
    del Ambiente (CEPIS)
Casilla 4337
Lima 100
Peru

WHO Collaborating Centre for Environmental and Epidemiological
    Aspects of Diarrhoeal Diseases
Department of Epidemiology and Population Sciences
London School of Hygiene and Tropical Medicine
Keppel Street
London WC1E 7HT
England

WHO Collaborating Centre for Water Quality and Human Health
Robens Institute
University of Surrey
Guildford
Surrey GU2 5XH
England
    or
Community Water Supply and Sanitation
World Health Organization
1211 Geneva 27
Switzerland

Street food-vendors and restaurants may pose a special risk during an epidemic. Environmental health workers, or their equivalent, must be especially vigilant in inspecting food-handling practices. They should be given the authority to stop street sales or close restaurants when their inspections reveal insanitary practices.

Houseflies play a relatively small role in spreading cholera, but their presence in large numbers indicates poor sanitary conditions which favour transmission of the disease.

4
Being prepared
for a cholera epidemic

A strong programme for the control of diarrhoeal diseases (CDD) is the best preparation for a cholera epidemic, both in areas that have not yet been affected and in areas where seasonal recurrence of the disease may be expected. In the long term, improvements in the water supply and in sanitation are the best means of preventing cholera. In an outbreak, however, the best control measures are the early detection and treatment of people with cholera, and health education.

In an unprepared community, cholera can cause death in as many as 50% of severe cases. However, where health facilities are well organized, with trained staff and essential supplies, fatalities among patients presenting for treatment may be less than 1%. Sections 4.1 to 4.3 outline the elements that are considered to be of paramount importance if a national CDD programme is to be adequately prepared to control an outbreak of cholera.

4.1 Training in clinical management of patients with acute diarrhoea

In an active national CDD programme, medical and paramedical personnel receive intensive and continuing training to ensure that they are familiar with the most effective techniques for management of patients with acute diarrhoea, including cholera. WHO provides materials for clinical management training, which emphasize practice in assessing and treating patients with diarrhoea.[1]

---

[1] *Diarrhoea management training course: guidelines for conducting clinical training courses at health centres and small hospitals.* Geneva, World Health Organization, 1990 (unpublished WHO document CDD/SER/90.2, available on request from Programme for Control of Diarrhoeal Diseases, World Health Organization, 1211 Geneva 27, Switzerland).

The assessment and treatment procedures for cholera are essentially the same as for diarrhoea from other causes (see Annex 2).

4.2 Emergency stocks of essential supplies

In order to respond quickly to an epidemic of cholera and to prevent deaths from the disease, health facilities must have access to adequate quantities of essential supplies, particularly oral rehydration salts, intravenous fluids, and appropriate antibiotics.

During a cholera epidemic, these supplies may be suddenly needed in greater quantities than normal. To prepare for an outbreak, it is therefore essential to maintain additional stocks at appropriate points in the drug delivery system. Small "buffer stocks" may be placed at local health facilities, larger buffer stocks at district or provincial levels, and an adequate emergency stock at a central distribution point.

The buffer stocks are *additional* to the supplies needed to meet normal demands: they are not specifically set aside for a cholera outbreak, but they allow the distribution system to absorb sudden increases in the demand for specific supplies. The buffer stocks are put into the normal delivery system so that stocks are rotated sufficiently often to avoid their becoming outdated. (For guidance in estimating required supplies, see section 5.4.)

4.3 Surveillance and reporting

An adequate disease surveillance system facilitates the early detection of cholera, especially when daily records are maintained of diarrhoea cases seen in health facilities and by health workers in the community. *A cholera outbreak should be suspected if*:

- a patient older than 5 years develops severe dehydration or dies from acute watery diarrhoea; or
- there is a sudden increase in the daily number of patients with acute watery diarrhoea, especially patients who pass the "rice water" stools typical of cholera.

When such changes in the pattern of diarrhoea occur, health workers should immediately notify the nearest referral facility or the designated local health officer, if possible by telephone or radio. They should specify the name, address, and age of each patient, and the date the illness began. Members of voluntary organizations, religious leaders, students, and other community members can also be encouraged to help in detecting and reporting cases.

When this information comes from an area where cholera has not previously been confirmed, bacteriological and epidemiological investigations should be promptly arranged to determine the cause of the outbreak. The manager of the national CDD programme or the epidemic control unit should be informed immediately, so that appropriate control measures can be initiated.

5
Early responses to the threat of an outbreak

Countries with fully established CDD programmes have trained health professionals, disease surveillance systems, rehydration and other treatment supplies in health facilities, and continuing health education activities. Programmes in various government ministries and departments work together to improve water supply, sanitation, and food safety practices. When a cholera outbreak occurs, these activities need to be reinforced and applied to control of the disease. If measures to control cholera and other types of diarrhoea are not yet established, efforts must be made to implement them. In addition, the activities outlined in sections 5.1 to 5.5 should be initiated.

5.1 Notification according to International Health Regulations

Under the terms of the International Health Regulations of 1969,[1] cholera is one of three diseases for which it is mandatory to notify the World Health Organization. National health authorities should report the first *suspected* cases of cholera on their territory to WHO as rapidly as possible. Laboratory confirmation should be obtained at the earliest opportunity and also reported to WHO.

Health authorities in countries where cholera is *confirmed* should make a weekly report to WHO, containing — as a minimum — the numbers of new cases and deaths since the last report and the cumulative totals for the current year, recorded by region or other suitable geographical division. Information on the age distribution of cases and the number admitted to hospital is

---

[1] *International Health Regulations (1969)*, 3rd ed. Geneva, World Health Organization, 1983.

Box 7. Definition of cholera cases for international reporting

A case of cholera should be suspected when:

- in an area where the disease is not known to be present, a patient aged 5 years or more develops severe dehydration or dies from acute watery diarrhoea;

- in an area where there is a cholera epidemic, a patient aged 5 years or more[1] develops acute watery diarrhoea, with or without vomiting.

A case of cholera is confirmed when:

- *Vibrio cholerae* O1 is isolated from any patient with diarrhoea.

---

[1] For *management* of cases of acute watery diarrhoea in an area where there is a cholera epidemic, cholera should be suspected in all patients aged *2 years or more*. However, the inclusion of all cases of acute watery diarrhoea in the 2–4 year age group in the reporting of cholera greatly reduces the specificity of reporting.

---

also desirable. This information should be sent simultaneously to the appropriate WHO Regional Office and to WHO Headquarters in Geneva (telex 415 416 or telefax 41.22.791 07 46, attention: EPIDNATIONS).

When cholera is newly suspected in an area, the International Health Regulations require that the diagnosis should be confirmed by laboratory investigations as soon as possible. Once the presence of cholera in an area has been confirmed, it becomes unnecessary to confirm all subsequent cases. Neither the treatment nor the notification of suspected cases of cholera requires laboratory confirmation of the presence of *Vibrio cholerae* O1. Monitoring of an epidemic should, however, include laboratory confirmation of a small proportion of cases on a continuing basis.

Unfortunately, some countries do not report cases for fear that restrictions may be imposed on exports and on travel by their citizens, or that tourism may be affected. Officials reluctant to report cases should bear in mind that notification often facilitates negotiations for removing trade and travel restrictions, and promotes international collaboration in the control of cholera.

5.2 National coordinating committee

A national CDD programme, coordinated by a programme manager, is usually responsible for activities related to cholera control. The far-reaching effects of a cholera epidemic often also call for a national coordinating committee, reinforced by senior members from other relevant departments and ministries, to ensure full collaboration among the involved sectors and the rapid execution of control activities. This committee functions as a national cholera control committee, responsible for:

- epidemic preparedness;
- coordination among sectors;
- regional and international collaboration;
- collection and reporting of information on cholera cases and deaths;
- organization of any necessary special training;
- procurement, storage, and distribution of required supplies; and
- implementation, supervision, monitoring, and evaluation of control activities.

Depending on the size of the country and on its health service structure, similar committees may be created at sub-national or more peripheral levels.

Alternatively, some countries may have a national health emergency committee, which is responsible for controlling all epidemics and other health emergencies. The manager of the national CDD programme should be a member of this committee in order to facilitate the coordination of activities required for cholera control.

In the event that no such committees exist when a cholera outbreak threatens, an interministerial committee or special task force, with appropriate decision-making authority, should quickly be formed to carry out the coordinating functions described above.

5.3 Mobile control teams

If a cholera outbreak occurs or threatens in countries or areas where the peripheral health services are inadequate or have no experience in controlling the disease, mobile teams may need to be formed at the national, provincial, or district level, and be trained to:

- establish and operate temporary treatment centres;
- provide on-the-spot training in case management for local health staff;
- supervise appropriate environmental sanitary measures and disinfection;
- carry out health education activities and disseminate information to the public to prevent panic;
- arrange for an epidemiological study to establish, if possible, the mode of disease transmission involved in the outbreak;
- collect stool and environmental specimens, including suspected foods, for submission to a bacteriology laboratory; and
- provide the required emergency logistic support, such as delivery of supplies, to health facilities and laboratories.

The members of each team — who may be otherwise employed in public health services, hospitals, laboratories, or elsewhere — should be brought together for briefing on emergency activities, their individual responsibilities, the location of their supplies, and the situations in which the teams' services would be needed.

5.4 Supplies and equipment

Buffer and emergency stocks of essential supplies should already be in place before an epidemic starts (see section 4.2). It is important to establish a system to monitor their use and ensure their prompt replacement. Emergency supply requirements should be determined and individuals assigned to coordinate their procurement and distribution. The national coordinating committee or task force is responsible for controlling the provision of supplies and equipment by external agencies, if necessary, to ensure that all drugs and materials meet national standards and requirements, and to avoid duplication of requests. A single central system for recording all incoming supplies and their distribution to different parts of the country is desirable.

The supplies and equipment needed for 100 cases of cholera are listed in Box 8. To estimate the number of cases that can be expected in a country or area affected by a cholera epidemic, an attack rate of 0.2% can be used (i.e. 200 cases may be expected to occur in a population of 100 000). In a severe epidemic, the national attack rate may be 1.0% or higher, and may reach 10–20% in some

Box 8. Estimated minimum supplies needed to treat 100 patients during a cholera outbreak

Rehydration supplies[1]

- 650 packets oral rehydration salts (for 1 litre each)
- 120 bags Ringer's lactate solution,[2] 1 litre, with giving sets
- 10 scalp-vein sets
- 3 nasogastric tubes, 5.3 mm OD, 3.5 mm ID (16 French), 50 cm long, for adults
- 3 nasogastric tubes, 2.7 mm OD, 1.5 mm ID (8 French), 38 cm long, for children

Antibiotics

For adults:

- 60 capsules doxycycline, 100 mg (3 capsules per severely dehydrated patient)

or

- 480 capsules tetracycline, 250 mg (24 capsules per severely dehydrated patient)

For children:

- 300 tablets trimethoprim–sulfamethoxazole, TMP 20 mg + SMX 100 mg (15 tablets per severely dehydrated patient)

If selective chemoprophylaxis is planned, the additional requirements for four close contacts per severely dehydrated patient (about 80 people) are:

- 240 capsules doxycycline, 100 mg (3 capsules per person)

or

- 1920 capsules tetracycline, 250 mg (24 capsules per person)

Other treatment supplies

- 2 large water dispensers with tap (marked at 5- and 10-litre levels) for making ORS solution in bulk
- 20 bottles (1 litre) for oral rehydration solution (e.g. empty IV bottles)
- 20 bottles (0.5 litre) for oral rehydration solution
- 40 tumblers, 200 ml
- 20 teaspoons
- 5 kg cotton wool
- 3 reels adhesive tape

---

[1] The supplies listed are sufficient for intravenous fluid followed by oral rehydration salts for 20 severely dehydrated patients, and for oral rehy-dration salts alone for the other 80 patients.

[2] If Ringer's lactate solution is unavailable, normal saline may be substituted.

areas. However, calculations based on an attack rate of 0.2% should allow enough supplies to meet needs during the first weeks of the epidemic, during which time the requirements can be reassessed.

5.5 Emergency treatment centres

Simplified treatment is the most important advance in cholera control and means that effective treatment can be within the immediate reach of most patients. Many deaths can thus be prevented, and the excellent results obtained also serve to calm public fears.

Most cases can be treated in existing health centres if rehydration materials (oral rehydration salts and intravenous fluid) and antibiotics are available, and health workers are trained in the management of diarrhoea.

If appropriate facilities, supplies, and trained staff are unavailable or are far away, or if there are too many cases to be handled by existing facilities, it will be necessary to establish emergency treatment facilities in affected communities. Temporary facilities can be established in huts, school buildings, or tents, and can be provided with the necessary supplies and trained staff.

These facilities, set up to provide rapid and efficient treatment for a large number of patients, should *not* be used to quarantine them: quarantine does not help to control the epidemic. Furthermore, while it is advisable to restrict contact between patients and the surrounding community to a minimum, it is *not* necessary to apply strict isolation measures, such as face masks, gloves, or special clothing for health staff and visiting family members. As in any unit treating patients with a communicable disease, it is important to have convenient hand-washing facilities for people working with and visiting cholera patients. The safe disposal of excreta and vomit is essential (see section 7.2).

6
Management
of the patient with cholera

Prompt recognition of cholera cases is important in order to start treatment as early as possible and to reduce potential contamination of the environment. *Cholera should be suspected when*:

- a patient older than 5 years develops severe dehydration from acute watery diarrhoea (usually with vomiting); or
- *any* patient older than 2 years has acute watery diarrhoea *in an area where there is an outbreak of cholera*.

Early case recognition also permits infected household contacts to be identified and helps the epidemiologist to investigate how cholera is being spread so that specific control measures can be implemented.

Patients must be treated as rapidly as possible, to reduce the risk of shock. For this reason, all patients with cholera should seek treatment from a trained health worker. During epidemics, when there are many cases but few health workers, grouping cholera patients in a single centre can facilitate treatment and also help to reduce environmental contamination.

6.1 Rehydration therapy

The dehydration, acidosis, and potassium depletion typical of cholera result from the loss of water and salts through diarrhoea and vomiting. Rehydration therapy consists of replacing water and salts in the proportions lost. Because large volumes of fluid may be rapidly lost, frequent reassessment during and after rehydration is essential until the diarrhoea stops.

While preparing to go to a health facility for treatment, patients with cholera should immediately start increasing the amount of fluids they drink. Sugar–salt solution and other fluids available in the home, including water, can be used to prevent or delay the onset of dehydration on the way to the health facility. However, these measures are inadequate for *treating* dehydration caused by acute diarrhoea, particularly cholera, in which the stool loss and risks of shock are often high. Where available for use in the home, oral rehydration salts (ORS) solution can also be taken from the onset of diarrhoea.

At the health facility, 80–90% of cholera patients can usually be adequately treated with ORS solution alone, without intravenous therapy. The composition of ORS solution approximates the water and salts contained in the diarrhoeal stool. Prepackaged ORS is the most suitable product for use in remote areas; when supplies are scarce, ORS packets should be reserved for this purpose. In hospitals and health centres, where large volumes are consumed daily, ORS solution can be made from packets or by weighing out the individual ingredients in appropriate quantities for the required volumes. A rice-based ORS solution may also be prepared (see Box 9).

Patients with cholera require intravenous rehydration more often than patients with diarrhoea due to other causes. Even in cholera, however, intravenous electrolyte solutions should be used only for the initial rehydration of *severely dehydrated* patients, including those who are in shock. Ringer's lactate solution (Hartmann's solution for injection) is the preferred fluid for intravenous rehydration. Its composition is suitable for treating patients of all ages and with all types of diarrhoea. (Some specially prepared poly-electrolyte solutions are also suitable, but are less widely available.)

Normal saline solution is somewhat less effective for intravenous rehydration, but can be used if Ringer's lactate solution is unavailable. *Plain glucose solutions are ineffective and should not be used.*

Cholera patients started on intravenous therapy should be given ORS solution as soon as they can drink, even before the initial intravenous therapy has been completed. They should then be treated with ORS solution until diarrhoea stops. After rehydration, patients should also be permitted to drink water.

For further information on rehydration therapy, see Annex 2.

6.2 Feeding the cholera patient

Food should be given after 3–4 hours of treatment, when rehydration is completed. Breast-feeding of infants and young children should be continued.

Box 9. To make 10 litres of ORS solution from bulk ingredients[1]

In 10 litres of water, completely dissolve the sugar and salts in the amounts shown below. Use the usual drinking-water. Boiled water, cooled before use, or chlorinated water is best. If larger volumes are prepared, the amount of each ingredient should be increased proportionally. ORS solution should be used within 24 hours; after that time, unused solution should be discarded and fresh solution prepared.

---

sodium chloride (common salt)	35 grams
plus	
glucose, anhydrous	200 grams
or	
sucrose (common sugar)	400 grams
or	
glucose, monohydrate	220 grams
plus	
trisodium citrate, dihydrate	29 grams
or	
sodium bicarbonate	25 grams
plus	
potassium chloride	15 grams

---

[1] To make 10 litres of *rice-based ORS solution*, boil 500 grams of rice powder in 11 litres of water for 5 minutes. (The extra litre allows for water lost during boiling.) Cool the liquid. Add 35 grams sodium chloride, 29 grams trisodium citrate (or 25 grams sodium bicarbonate), and 15 grams potassium chloride. Mix well. Rice-based ORS solution should be used within 8–12 hours, after which fresh solution should be prepared.

6.3 Antibiotics

In severe cases of cholera, antibiotics can reduce the volume and duration of diarrhoea, and shorten the period during which cholera vibrios are excreted. They can be given orally as soon as vomiting stops, usually within 3–4 hours after starting rehydration. There is no advantage in using injectable antibiotics, which are expensive.

The patients who benefit most from antibiotics are those who are severely dehydrated. Indiscriminate use of antibiotics in mild cases can quickly use up supplies and hasten the development of antibiotic resistance among cholera vibrios.

For adult cholera patients, doxycycline, a long-acting form of tetracycline, is the preferred antibiotic because only a single dose is needed. For children, paediatric tablets or liquid preparations of trimethoprim–sulfamethoxazole (TMP–SMX) are recommended. A single dose of doxycycline has not yet been shown to be effective in children. Tetracycline, however, is effective in children but in some countries is not available for paediatric use. Furazolidone, erythromycin, and chloramphenicol are other effective alternatives for adults and children. (See Table 3 of Annex 2 for antibiotics used in treating severe cholera.)

Sulfadoxine is not effective, and should not be used. A single dose can cause serious and even fatal reactions.

The choice of antibiotic should take into account local patterns of resistance to antibiotics. Knowledge of antibiotic sensitivity patterns of recent isolates in the immediate area or in adjacent areas is therefore important. Antibiotic-resistant *Vibrio cholerae* O1 should be suspected if diarrhoea continues after 48 hours of antibiotic treatment.

No antidiarrhoeal, anti-emetic, antispasmodic, cardiotonic, or corticosteroid drugs should be used to treat cholera. Blood transfusions and plasma volume expanders are not necessary.

7
Preventing the spread of an outbreak

People contract cholera from drinking water or eating food contaminated with cholera organisms. Prevention is based on reducing the chances of ingesting vibrios. When cholera appears in a community, efforts must be intensified to promote the sanitary disposal of human waste, the provision of safe water, and safe practices in handling food (see section 3). In addition, the measures described in sections 7.1 to 7.3 should be implemented.

7.1 Health education

Health education is the key to public awareness and cooperation. An outbreak can be more quickly controlled when people understand how to help limit its spread. Experienced health educators therefore play an important role in epidemic control. Community and service organizations can also be useful in disseminating health messages through their programmes.

It is particularly important to inform people that most cases of cholera can be treated with simple measures, and that vaccination is not effective. There is no substitute for drinking only safe water, practising good personal hygiene, and preparing food safely. (See Annex 3 for examples of appropriate health education messages.)

7.2 Disinfection and funeral precautions

In unhygienic living conditions, contamination of a cholera patient's surroundings is almost inevitable. A patient's bedding and clothing can be disinfected by stirring them for 5 minutes in boiling water. Bedding, including mattresses, can also be disinfected by thorough drying in the sun. Moreover, in order to minimize contamination of the washing area, the patient's

---

Box 10. Key points for public education about cholera

To prevent cholera

- Drink only water from a safe source or water that has been disinfected (boiled or chlorinated).
- Cook food or reheat it thoroughly, and eat it while it is still hot.
- Avoid uncooked food unless it can be peeled or shelled.
- Wash your hands after any contact with excreta and before preparing or eating food.
- Dispose of human excreta promptly and safely.

Remember

- With proper treatment, cholera is not fatal.
- Take patients with suspected cholera immediately to a health worker for treatment.
- Give increased quantities of fluids (if available, oral rehydration salts solution) as soon as diarrhoea starts.
- Cholera vaccination is *not* recommended.

---

clothing and other articles can be disinfected by drying them in the sun before washing.

Appropriate treatment of cholera stools also helps to control the spread of an epidemic. The simplest method for a family or small rural health unit to dispose of cholera stools is by putting them in a pit latrine or by burying them.

In larger health facilities, safe treatment and disposal of liquid waste from cholera patients, including excreta and vomit, can be accomplished by sterilization or burial. Stools and vomit from cholera patients can be mixed with disinfectants (e.g. cresol). Hospitals can use a prepared acid solution to mix with the waste to lower it to a pH below 4.5. After 15 minutes it is generally safe to dispose of this mixture in a toilet or latrine, or by burying it.

Excessive quantities of acid should not be used to lower the pH more than necessary. Furthermore, the toilet and other installations must be corrosion-resistant (e.g. made of ceramic material), or extensive damage to the sewage system can result. Acid should not be used when hospital sewage is drained to a septic tank, because it will interfere with and damage the functioning of the tank.

The preferred method for disposing of semisolid waste is incineration, provided that the incinerator used is designed to destroy contaminated waste. Semisolid waste from cholera patients should be kept separate from other kinds of waste and, if possible, put into single-use, moisture-proof bags. If the waste is transported from its initial storage point to an on-site incinerator by means of handcarts, this equipment must be cleaned regularly and used only for transporting waste. The bags used to gather and carry the waste should also be burned. If the waste is transferred for treatment outside the health facility, the transport vehicle should have an enclosed, leak-proof body, which should be cleaned after each use and disinfected regularly.

Box 11. Some public health supply requirements

- Disinfectant (e.g. cresol)
- Muriatic acid
- pH testing kits
- Chlorine chemicals for water treatment (gas chlorine, sodium hypochlorite, calcium hypochlorite, bleaching powder, and chlorine tablets)
- DPD (diethyl-p-phenylenediamine) water testing kits for measuring residual chlorine levels

---

Funerals for people who die of cholera — or of any other cause in a community affected by cholera — can contribute to the spread of an epidemic. Funerals may bring people from uninfected areas into an infected area from which they can carry the cholera organism back home. It is therefore important to make every effort, through intensive health education or by legislation, to limit funeral gatherings, ritual washing of the dead, or funeral feasts. To reduce the spread of infection, funerals should be held quickly and near the place of death.

Those who care for and clean up after the cholera patient, and especially those who prepare the body (which may include cleaning the large bowel), can be exposed to high concentrations of vibrios. These are often the same people who then prepare large quantities of food for others who attend the funeral. Discouraging these practices can substantially reduce the risk of the transmission of infection. If funeral feasts cannot be cancelled, and if other people are not available to prepare the food, meticulous handwashing with soap and clean water is essential before food is handled. A designated health worker, present at the funeral gathering, can be helpful in supervising the use of hygienic practices.

7.3 Ineffective control measures

Efforts to control cholera through mass chemoprophylaxis, vaccination, and travel and trade restrictions are ineffective. When cholera threatens, however, pressure to use these measures may come from a frightened public or from uninformed officials. National policies on appropriate control measures are therefore vital and should be developed before an outbreak occurs.

7.3.1 Chemoprophylaxis

Treatment of an entire community with antibiotics, referred to as *mass chemoprophylaxis,* has never succeeded in limiting the spread of cholera. There are a number of reasons for this failure:

- It usually takes longer to organize distribution of the drug than for the infection to spread.
- The effect of the drug persists for only a day or two, after which reinfection can occur.
- To prevent reinfection, the entire population would need to be treated simultaneously and then isolated.
- It may be difficult to persuade people who are symptom-free to take a drug.

Mass chemoprophylaxis not only fails to prevent the spread of cholera, but also diverts attention and resources from effective measures. In several countries, it has also contributed to the emergence of antibiotic resistance in the vibrio, depriving severely ill patients of a valuable treatment.

Selective chemoprophylaxis may be useful for members of a household, who share food and shelter with a cholera patient. However, in an outbreak of El Tor cholera, secondary cases may be unusual. Moreover, in societies where intimate social mixing and the exchange of food between households are common, it is difficult to determine who is a close contact.

The value of selective chemoprophylaxis thus depends on local circumstances. It is justified only if surveillance shows that the secondary attack rate in the community is high, i.e. that an average of at least one household member in five becomes ill after the first case occurs in the household.

If selective chemoprophylaxis is used, it should be given to all close contacts as soon as possible after the initial case is recognized. The prophylactic dose of antibiotic is the same as the therapeutic dose (see Annex 2). Doxycycline is preferred because only a single dose is needed.

7.3.2 Vaccination

For a number of reasons, the vaccine currently available is of no help in controlling cholera. Field trials have shown that:

- the vaccine frequently lacks the required potency;
- even when potent, the vaccine is not very effective — that is, not all persons who are vaccinated are protected;
- any protection that does occur lasts for only 3–6 months; and
- vaccination does not reduce the incidence of asymptomatic infections or prevent the spread of infection.

In addition, vaccination can give a false sense of security to people who have been vaccinated and to health authorities, who may then neglect more effective measures. Vaccination campaigns divert resources and manpower from more useful control activities.

Because of the limitations of cholera vaccination, the Twenty-sixth World Health Assembly (1973) abolished the requirement in the International Health Regulations for a certificate of vaccination against cholera. No country currently requires travellers to have a cholera vaccination certificate.

7.3.3 Travel and trade restrictions *(cordon sanitaire)*

Travel and trade restrictions between countries or different areas within a country do not prevent the spread of cholera. Even the most concentrated efforts cannot detect and isolate all infected travellers, most of whom have no signs of illness. Moreover, a *cordon sanitaire* requires check-posts to be set up and movements to be restricted. These activities divert substantial human and other resources from more effective control measures.

As well as being ineffective, restrictions on travel and trade severely disrupt the economy of a country or area and, as a result, encourage the suppression of information regarding cholera outbreaks. Collaboration between local, national, and international authorities in their joint efforts to control cholera outbreaks may thus be severely hampered.

Box 12. Risk of cholera transmission through food trade[1]

Vibrio cholerae O1 can survive on a variety of foodstuffs for up to 5 days at ambient temperature and up to 10 days at $5-10\,^{\circ}C$. The organism can also survive freezing. Low temperatures, however, limit proliferation of the organism and thus may prevent the level of contamination from reaching an infective dose.

The cholera vibrio is sensitive to acidity and drying, and commercially prepared acidic (pH 4.5 or less) or dried foods are therefore without risk. Gamma irradiation and temperatures above $70\,^{\circ}C$ also destroy the vibrio, and foods processed by these methods, according to the standards of the Codex Alimentarius, are safe unless subsequently contaminated.

The foods that cause greatest concern to importing countries are seafood and vegetables that may be consumed raw. Cases of cholera have occurred as a result of eating food, usually seafood, transported across international borders by individuals.

However, a large number of tests carried out on commercially imported foods from affected countries (most recently from South America) have not detected *Vibrio cholerae* O1. Indeed, although individual cases and clusters of cases have been reported, WHO has not documented a significant outbreak of cholera resulting from commercially imported food.

In summary, although there is a theoretical risk of cholera transmission associated with international food trade, the weight of evidence suggests that this risk is small and can normally be dealt with by means other than an embargo on importation.

---

[1] Adapted from a Statement by the Global Task Force on Cholera Control to the 44th World Health Assembly (10 May 1991)

8
Epidemiology: investigating an outbreak

At the start of a cholera outbreak, even as general control measures are applied, epidemiological studies can determine the magnitude of the outbreak and the mode of transmission, so that more specific and effective control measures can be applied. Recording the time and place of suspected and confirmed cases, preferably on a spot map, can help identify sources and routes of infection.

Case-control studies, although difficult to conduct and interpret, may help to define the mode of transmission, particularly in newly affected areas. Countries may request assistance from WHO or other outside sources to conduct them. Laboratory analysis of samples of suspect water, sewage, and food may also be helpful.

During cholera outbreaks in newly affected areas, people of all ages may contract the disease. However, the more mobile members of the community (usually adults) are more frequently affected because of their greater exposure to possible sources of contamination, such as food or drinks taken outside the home. In contrast, a preponderance of cases in children suggests that the disease is endemic in the area.

9
The role of the laboratory

Successful treatment of cholera does not depend on the results of laboratory examinations. However, laboratory analysis of specimens from the first suspected cases *is* essential to confirm the presence of cholera and determine the characteristics of the organism; control measures can then be implemented.

A sufficient number of stool specimens should be examined to identify the causative organism and test its sensitivity to antibiotics. Once the presence of cholera is confirmed, it is not necessary to examine specimens from all cases or contacts. In fact, this should be discouraged since it places an unnecessary burden on laboratory facilities and is not required for effective treatment.

Box 13. Diagnostic laboratory supplies for presumptive identification of *Vibrio cholerae* O1 at a peripheral laboratory

100 rectal swabs
500 g Cary-Blair medium
3 x 300 g TCBS medium
or
    250 g trypticase
    250 g sodium taurocholate
    2 x 250 g gelatin
    25 g potassium tellurite
25 g sodium desoxycholate
5 g tetramethyl-*p*-phenylenediamine hydrochloride
250 g Kligler's iron agar
500 g nutrient agar
5 x 2 ml polyvalent O-group 1 cholera diagnostic antiserum
1 kg Bacto-peptone culture medium
500 Petri dishes (9 cm)
1000 test-tubes (13 x 100 mm)
1000 disposable Bijou bottles

Environmental sampling, including the use of Moore swabs for night-soil and sewage samples, can help clarify how infection is being spread.

Local laboratories that normally undertake bacteriological cultures should be capable of culturing and identifying *Vibrio cholerae* O1, using the methods outlined in Annex 5. They should stock the necessary supplies of media and antisera, and be able to provide transport media and rectal swabs to the fieldworkers who will collect the specimens.

The laboratory must keep clinicians and epidemiologists promptly informed of all results. National laboratories may contact WHO to arrange for technical cooperation with reference laboratories, for example to verify laboratory findings or to characterize an atypical strain.

9.1 Handling of stool samples

Stool specimens or rectal swabs from suspected cases should be promptly submitted for laboratory examination in a transport medium (e.g. Cary-Blair medium), a supply of which should be stocked by the local health centre or health officer. (Techniques for collecting specimens are described in Annex 5.) If a transport medium is not available, a cotton-tipped rectal swab can be soaked in the liquid stool, placed in a sterile plastic bag, tightly sealed, and sent to the laboratory. Ideally, specimens should be collected before any antibiotics are given to the patients.

The name, age, and address of the patient, the main clinical signs, and the date and time when the specimen was obtained should be written on a request slip and sent with each specimen.

9.2 Reference laboratory

In areas at risk, a national reference laboratory should be assigned the responsibility for providing culture media and essential antisera, training workers in local and regional laboratories in appropriate isolation techniques, and monitoring the quality of laboratory services.

The reference laboratory should be able to identify, biotype, and serotype *Vibrio cholerae* O1, and perform antibiotic sensitivity testing. For more complicated procedures (e.g. phage typing and toxin testing), it may refer to an appropriate international reference laboratory.

Box 14. Some International Reference Laboratories

The following centres have facilities for isolating and identifying *Vibrio cholerae* O1, enterotoxin testing, phage typing, and ribotyping. Training in the laboratory diagnosis of enteropathogens, including cholera, and other technical assistance can be arranged. The centre should be consulted before strains are sent.

WHO Collaborating Centre for Research, Training
and Control in Diarrhoeal Diseases
International Centre for Diarrhoeal Disease Research,
Bangladesh (ICDDR,B)
G.P.O. Box 128
Dhaka 100
Bangladesh

WHO Collaborating Centre for Diarrhoeal Diseases
Research and Training
National Institute of Cholera and Enteric Diseases
P-33, CIT Road Scheme XM
Beliaghata
P.O. Box 177
Calcutta 700 016
India

WHO Collaborating Centre for Phage-Typing and
Resistance of Enterobacteria
Central Public Health Laboratory
61 Colindale Avenue
London NW9 5HT
England

Division of Bacterial Diseases
Enteric Disease Branch
Center for Infectious Diseases
Centers for Disease Control
Atlanta
GA 30333
USA

10
After an outbreak

As an outbreak of cholera subsides, emphasis should shift from emergency control measures to preparedness for future outbreaks and long-term efforts to improve the safety of public water supplies and sanitation facilities.

Public health education programmes must continually stress the principles of good personal hygiene, and the importance of using only safe water, of the safe disposal of excreta, and of safe food practices.

Ideally, a water supply system in urban areas should provide potable water under constant positive pressure through a system piped into private homes. The water should be treated with an effective chemical such as chlorine. Properly operated facilities for disposing of excreta in all households are a goal towards which all local authorities should strive.

In rural areas, water sources should be protected from surface contamination, and latrines should always be situated so as to drain away from water sources and catchment areas. The installation of simple devices such as tube wells should be encouraged.

Cholera will ultimately be brought under control only when water supplies, sanitation, personal hygiene, and food handling practices are safe enough to prevent the transmission of *Vibrio cholerae* O1.

Additional information on cholera control

Unless otherwise noted, the publications below are available in English only.

A guide on food safety for travellers. Geneva, World Health Organization, 1991 (unpublished WHO document WHO/FOS/91.1).

This leaflet describes what travellers should do to avoid illnesses caused by unsafe food and drink, and what to do if they get diarrhoea. Available from Distribution and Sales, World Health Organization, 1211 Geneva 27, Switzerland.

- Arabic, English, French, German, Spanish (Chinese, Italian, Japanese versions in preparation).

Cholera — basic facts for travellers. Geneva, World Health Organization, 1992 (unpublished WHO document).

This leaflet is aimed at those travelling to countries where cholera occurs. It explains what cholera is and how, through simple precautions, it can be avoided. Available from Distribution and Sales, World Health Organization, 1211 Geneva 27, Switzerland.

- English, French, Spanish.

Cairncross S. *Small scale sanitation.* London, London School of Hygiene and Tropical Medicine, 1988.

This text provides detailed and illustrated instructions for building basic latrines and water supply systems for families and small communities. It is written especially for community health workers and others with no training in this technical area.

Diarrhoea management training course: guidelines for conducting clinical training courses at health centres and small hospitals. Geneva, World Health Organization, 1990 (unpublished WHO document CDD/SER/90.2).

This training package includes a Participant Manual, Instructor Guide, a set of slides, and a video tape for use in a 3–4 day training course in diarrhoea case management for physicians, nurses, and other health workers. Participants learn through written exercises, drills, and practical experience how to assess and treat patients with diarrhoea, including cholera. The course can be conducted in a health facility wherever there are sufficient numbers of diarrhoea patients available for the practical training. Because no special facilities are required, it is ideal for training health workers in the field and, where a cholera epidemic threatens, for training those responsible for establishing emergency treatment facilities. Available on request from the Programme for Control of Diarrhoeal Diseases, World Health Organization, 1211 Geneva 27, Switzerland.

- English, French.

Fact sheets on environmental sanitation for cholera control. Geneva, World Health Organization (in preparation.)

Fact sheets on appropriate measures to improve environmental sanitation for prevention of cholera epidemics. The emphasis is on the interventions that will result in the best use of existing facilities, and on disinfection of water. Information from several technical manuals is brought together in a set of brief, easy-to-use instructions. Will be available on request from Community Water Supply and Sanitation, World Health Organization, 1211 Geneva 27, Switzerland.

Guidelines for drinking-water quality, Vols 1–3. Geneva, World Health Organization, 1984–1985.

The guidelines include: Vol. 1, Recommendations; Vol. 2, Health criteria and other supporting information; Vol. 3, Drinking-water control in small-community supplies. They are intended for use by countries as a basis for the development of standards to ensure the safety of drinking-water supplies. (Second edition in preparation.)

- Arabic, Chinese, English, French, Russian.

Management of the patient with cholera. Geneva, World Health Organization, 1991 (unpublished WHO document WHO/CDD/SER/91.15 Rev 1).

This document is reproduced in Annex 2. It is also available on request from the Programme for Control of Diarrhoeal Diseases, World Health Organization, 1211 Geneva 27, Switzerland.

- English, French, Spanish (Portuguese version in preparation).

Management of the patient with diarrhoea: supervisory skills course. Geneva, World Health Organization, 1990 (unpublished WHO document).

This training module is designed for use in courses for supervisors of health workers. It uses written exercises and case examples to present elements of the management of patients with diarrhoea, including cholera. Available on request from the Programme for Control of Diarrhoeal Diseases, World Health Organization, 1211 Geneva 27, Switzerland.

- English, French, Spanish.

Manual for laboratory investigations of acute enteric infections. Geneva, World Health Organization, 1987 (unpublished WHO document CDD/83.3 Rev 1).

Available on request from the Programme for Control of Diarrhoeal Diseases , World Health Organization, 1211 Geneva 27, Switzerland.

- English, French.

Rajagopalan S, Schiffman MA. *Guide to simple sanitary measures for the control of enteric diseases.* Geneva, World Health Organization, 1974.

Instructions for building latrines and simple water supply systems, including information that would be especially useful under emergency conditions in hospitals, schools, and refugee camps. A chapter on food sanitation provides guidelines for safe handling of food during its production, processing, and preparation for consumption. Tables identify the chemicals needed by those responsible for chlorinating water and disinfecting contaminated articles.

Franceys R, Pickford J, Reed R. *A guide to the development of on-site sanitation.* Geneva, World Health Organization, 1992.

This publication describes all practical options for on-site sanitation, that is, means for dealing with excreta where they are deposited rather than through sewerage systems. It outlines the foundations of sanitary practice and provides details on the design, construction, and maintenance of various types of latrines, privies, and septic tanks. The planning and development of on-site sanitation projects are addressed, and the book also includes references, selected further readings, and a useful glossary of terms.

- English (French and Spanish versions in preparation).

The treatment and prevention of acute diarrhoea: practical guidelines, 2nd ed. Geneva, World Health Organization, 1989.

This book is designed for use by community health workers to help them assess dehydration and treat patients with diarrhoea. It also contains ideas for encouraging practices that will help to prevent diarrhoea. (Third edition in preparation.)

- Chinese, English, French, Portuguese, Russian, Spanish.

Building a ventilated improved pit latrine[1]

A ventilated improved pit latrine is a practical means of disposing of human excreta and may be a good solution for use in rural areas. However, the decision on the type of latrine to be selected should take account of local factors such as type of soil and density of population.

The latrine must be constructed at least 30 metres away from a well or other source of drinking-water and, where possible, 6 metres away from a house. It should not be located uphill from the water source or dug in marshy soil.

A latrine 2 metres deep with an opening 1 metre x 1 metre can be used by a family of five for 2–4 years. (This assumes an accumulation rate of between 60 and 100 litres per person per year.) To keep bad odours and flies to a minimum, ventilation for this type of pit latrine is provided by an external vertical vent, topped by a fly screen. The edges of the pit are higher than ground level to prevent rain or other water from draining into it. The latrine should have a concrete or wooden slab which should reach to the walls of the superstructure. Where possible, concrete reinforced with steel wires at least 8 mm in diameter and 150 mm apart should be used because of its durability and resistance.

The slabs and floor should be washed clean daily and disinfected regularly with cresol or bleaching powder. After the pit is loaded to two-thirds of its capacity (1.3 metres height), it should be filled with soil and compacted, and a new pit should be dug.

---

[1] For more specific instructions see Cairncross S. *Small scale sanitation.* London, London School of Hygiene and Tropical Medicine, 1988.

Annex 2
Management of the patient with cholera

Cholera should be suspected when:

- a patient older than 5 years develops severe dehydration from acute watery diarrhoea (usually with vomiting); or
- any patient above the age of 2 years has acute watery diarrhoea *in an area where there is an outbreak of cholera.*

Steps in the management of suspected cholera

Step 1. Assess the patient for dehydration.

Step 2. Rehydrate the patient, and monitor frequently. Then re-assess hydration status.

Step 3. Maintain hydration: replace continuing fluid losses until diarrhoea stops.

Step 4. Give an oral antibiotic to the patient with severe dehydration.

Step 5. Feed the patient.

Step 1. Assess the patient for dehydration

Use Table 1 to determine whether the patient has:

- severe dehydration
- some dehydration
- no signs of dehydration.

Table 1. Assessment of the diarrhoea patient for dehydration[a]			
1. LOOK AT:			
CONDITION	Well, alert	*Restless, irritable*	*Lethargic or unconscious; floppy*
EYES	Normal	Sunken	Very sunken and dry
TEARS	Present	Absent	Absent
MOUTH and TONGUE	Moist	Dry	Very dry
THIRST	Drinks normally, not thirsty	*Thirsty, drinks eagerly*	*Drinks poorly or not able to drink*
2. FEEL:			
SKIN PINCH	Goes back quickly	*Goes back slowly*	*Goes back very slowly*
3. DECIDE:	The patient has **no signs of dehydration**	If the patient has **two or more signs,** including at least one *sign*, there is **some dehydration**	If the patient has **two or more signs, in-**cluding at least one *sign*, there is severe **dehydration**

[a] In adults and children older than 5 years, other *signs* for severe dehydration are *absent radial pulse* and *low blood pressure*. The skin pinch may be less useful in patients with marasmus (severe wasting) or kwashiorkor (severe malnutrition with oedema), or obese patients. Tears are a relevant sign only for infants and young children.

Step 2. Rehydrate the patient, and monitor frequently; reassess hydration status

For severe dehydration:

- *Give IV fluid* immediately to replace fluid deficit. Use Ringer's lactate solution or, if not available, normal saline.
- Start IV fluid immediately. If the patient can drink, begin giving oral rehydration salts (ORS) solution by mouth while the drip is being set up.

- *For patients aged 1 year and older*, give 100 ml/kg IV in 3 hours, as follows:

  — 30 ml/kg as rapidly as possible (within 30 minutes); then

  — 70 ml/kg in the next 2 ½ hours.

- *For patients aged less than 1 year*, give 100 ml/kg IV in 6 hours, as follows:

  — 30 ml/kg in the first hour; then

  — 70 ml/kg in the next 5 hours.

- *Monitor the patient* very frequently. After the initial 30 ml/kg have been given, the radial pulse should be strong (and blood pressure should be normal). If the pulse is not yet strong, continue to give IV fluid rapidly.

- *Give ORS solution* (about 5 ml/kg per hour) as soon as the patient can drink, in addition to IV fluid.

- *Reassess the patient* after 3 hours (infants after 6 hours), using Table 1:

  — If there are still signs of *severe dehydration* (this is rare), repeat the IV therapy.

  — If there are signs of *some dehydration*, continue as indicated below for some dehydration.

  — If there are *no signs of dehydration*, go on to Step 3 to maintain hydration by replacing continuing fluid losses.

For some dehydration:

- *Give ORS solution* in the amount recommended in Table 2. If the patient passes watery stools or wants more ORS solution than shown, give more.

- *Monitor the patient* frequently to ensure that ORS solution is taken satisfactorily and to detect patients with profuse and continuing diarrhoea who will require closer monitoring.

- *Reassess the patient* after 4 hours, using Table 1:

  — If signs of *severe dehydration* have appeared (this is rare), treat as in Step 1, above.

  — If there is still *some dehydration*, repeat the procedures for some dehydration, and start to offer food and other fluids.

  — If there are *no signs of dehydration*, go on to Step 3 to maintain hydration by replacing continuing fluid losses.

Age[a]	Less than 4 months	4–11 months	12–23 months	2–4 years	5–14 years	15 years or older
Table 2. Approximate amount of ORS solution to give in the first 4 hours						
Weight	Less than 5 kg	5–7.9 kg	8–10.9 kg	11–15.9 kg	16–29.9 kg	30 kg or more
ORS solution in ml	200–400	400–600	600–800	800–1200	1200–2200	2200–4000

[a] Use the patient's age only when you do not know the weight. The approximate amount of ORS required (in ml) can also be calculated by multiplying the patient's weight (in kg) by 75.

Notes on rehydration

Most patients absorb enough ORS solution to achieve rehydration even when they are vomiting. Vomiting usually subsides within 2–3 hours, as rehydration is achieved.

A nasogastric tube should be used for ORS solution if the patient has signs of some dehydration and cannot drink, or for severe dehydration *only* if IV therapy is not possible at the treatment facility.

Urine output decreases as dehydration develops, and may cease. It usually resumes within 6–8 hours after starting rehydration. Regular urinary output (every 3–4 hours) is a good sign that enough fluid is being given.

For no signs of dehydration:

Patients *first seen* with *no signs of dehydration* can be treated at home.

- *Give ORS packets* to take home. Give enough packets for 2 days. Demonstrate how to prepare and give the solution. The caregiver should give the patient the following amount of ORS solution:

Age	Amount of solution after each loose stool	ORS packets needed
Less than 24 months	50–100 ml	Enough for 500 ml/day
2–9 years	100–200 ml	Enough for 1000 ml/day
10 years or more	As much as wanted	Enough for 2000 ml/day

- *Instruct the patient or the care-giver to return* if the patient develops any of the following signs:
  - increased number of watery stools
  - eating or drinking poorly
  - marked thirst
  - repeated vomiting;

  or if any signs indicating other problems develop:
  - fever
  - blood in stool.

Step 3. Maintain hydration; replace continuing fluid losses until diarrhoea stops

When a patient who has been rehydrated with IV fluid or ORS solution is reassessed, and has *no signs of dehydration*, continue to give ORS solution to maintain normal hydration. The aim is to replace stool losses as they occur with an equivalent amount of ORS solution.

- *As a guide, give the patient:*

Age	Amount of solution, after each loose stool
Less than 24 months	100 ml
2–9 years	200 ml
10 years or more	As much as wanted

The amount of ORS solution actually required to maintain hydration varies greatly from patient to patient, depending on the volume of stool passed. The amount required is greatest in the first 24 hours of treatment, and is especially large in patients who present with severe dehydration. In the first 24 hours, such patients require an *average* of 200 ml of ORS solution per kg of body weight, but some may need as much as 350 ml/kg.

- *Continue to reassess the patient* for signs of dehydration at least every 4 hours to ensure that sufficient ORS solution is being taken. Patients with profuse continuing diarrhoea require more frequent monitoring. If signs of *some dehydration* are detected, the patient should be rehydrated as described on pages 42 and 43, before receiving treatment to maintain hydration.

A few patients, whose continuing stool output is very large, may have difficulty in drinking the volume of ORS needed to maintain hydration. If such patients become tired, vomit frequently, or develop abdominal distension, ORS solution should be stopped and hydration should be maintained intravenously with Ringer's lactate solution or normal saline; 50 ml/kg should be given in 3 hours. After this, it is usually possible to resume treatment with ORS solution.

- *Keep the patient under observation*, if possible, until diarrhoea stops, or is infrequent and of small volume. This is especially important for any patient who presented with severe dehydration.

If a patient must be discharged before diarrhoea has stopped, show the care-giver how to prepare and give ORS solution, and instruct him or her to continue to give ORS solution, as above. Also instruct the care-giver to bring the patient back if any of the signs listed on page 44 should develop.

Step 4. Give an oral antibiotic to the patient with severe dehydration

An effective antibiotic can reduce the volume of diarrhoea in patients with severe cholera and shorten the period during which *Vibrio cholerae* O1 is excreted. In addition, it will usually stop the diarrhoea within 48 hours, thus shortening the period of hospitalization.

- *Start antibiotics* after the patient has been rehydrated (usually in 4–6 hours), and vomiting has stopped.

There is no advantage in using injectable antibiotics, which are expensive. No other drugs should be used in the treatment of cholera.

Use Table 3 to select the antibiotic and dose.

Step 5. Feed the patient

- *Resume feeding* with a normal diet when vomiting has stopped.
- *Continue breast-feeding* infants and young children.

Table 3. Antibiotics used to treat cholera

Antibiotic[a]	Children	Adults
Doxycycline *a single dose*	—	300 mg[b]
Tetracycline *4 times per day* *for 3 days*	12.5 mg/kg	500 mg
Trimethoprim – sulfamethoxazole (TMP–SMX) *twice a day for 3 days*	TMP 5 mg/kg and SMX 25 mg/kg[c]	TMP 160 mg and SMX 800 mg
Furazolidone *4 times per day* *for 3 days*	1.25 mg/kg	100 mg[d]

[a] Erythromycin or chloramphenicol may be used when the antibiotics recommended are not available, or where *Vibrio cholerae* O1 is resistant to them.
[b] Doxycycline is the antibiotic of choice for adults (except pregnant women) because only one dose is required.
[c] TMP–SMX is the antibiotic of choice for children. Tetracycline is equally effective; however, in some countries it is not available for paediatric use.
[d] Furazolidone is the antibiotic of choice for pregnant women.

Complications

Pulmonary oedema is caused by giving *too much IV fluid*, especially when metabolic acidosis has not been corrected. The latter is most likely to occur when normal saline is used for IV rehydration and ORS solution is not given at the same time. When the guidelines for IV rehydration are followed, pulmonary oedema should not occur. ORS solution never causes pulmonary oedema.

Renal failure may occur when *too little IV fluid* is given, when shock is not rapidly corrected, or when shock is allowed to recur, especially in persons above the age of 60 years. Renal failure is rare when severe dehydration is rapidly corrected and normal hydration is maintained according to the guidelines.

Annex 3
Sample health education messages

The following sample messages may be adapted to local conditions and translated into local languages.

Three simple rules for cholera prevention

1. Cook your food
2. Boil your water
3. Wash your hands

Are you protected from cholera?
Do you prepare food safely?

Cooking kills cholera germs

- Thoroughly cook all meats, fish, and vegetables.
- Eat them while they are hot.

Washing protects from cholera

- Wash your *hands* before preparing or serving food.
- Wash your *dishes and utensils* with soap and water.
- Wash your *cutting board* especially well with soap and water.

Peeling protects from cholera

- Eat only fruits that have been freshly peeled, such as oranges and bananas.

Keep it clean — cook it, peel it, or leave it

Are you protected from cholera?
Is your water boiled or treated?

Even if it looks clean, water can contain cholera germs.

Water can be made safe in several ways:

- *Boiling* kills cholera germs: boil all drinking-water.

- *Chlorine* kills cholera germs: use 3 drops of *chlorine* solution in 1 litre of water. Mix well, and let it sit for half an hour before drinking.

To make the chlorine solution: mix 3 level tablespoons (33 grams) of bleaching powder in 1 litre of water.[1]

Drink safe water

[1] This quantity is for a bleaching powder that contains 30% concentration by weight of available chlorine. The quantity to be recommended must be adapted for the bleach available on the local market.

Are you protected from cholera?
Is your water stored safely?

Clean water can become contaminated again if it is not stored safely.

Water should be stored in a clean container with a small opening and a cover. It should be used within 24 hours.

Pour the water from the container — do not dip a cup into the container.

Keep it clean — store water safely

Are you protected from cholera?
Do you wash your hands?

Most dirt that causes cholera is invisible. It can be carried on hands without you knowing it.

Always wash your hands:

- after you use the toilet or latrine, or clean up your children
- before you prepare food
- before you eat and before you feed your children.

What is the best way to wash your hands?

- Always use soap or ash.
- Use plenty of clean water.
- Wash all parts of your hands — front, back, between the fingers, under the nails.

Keep it clean — wash your hands

Are you protected from cholera?
Do you use a toilet or latrine?

Cholera germs live in faeces. Even a person who is healthy may have cholera germs in the faeces.

Always use a toilet or latrine. If you don't have one — build one.

- Keep the toilet or latrine *clean.*
- Dispose of *babies'* faeces in the toilet or latrine (or bury them).
- *Wash your hands* with soap (or ash) and clean water after using the toilet or latrine.

Keep it clean — use a toilet or latrine

Are you prepared for cholera?
What should you do if you get it?

Cholera can be treated.

The biggest danger of cholera is loss of water from the body.
Don't panic — but *act quickly*.

- Drink oral rehydration salts (ORS) mixed with safe water (boiled or chlorinated).
- Go immediately to the health centre. Continue drinking as you go.

Now — before you or your family get cholera — find out where you can get ORS and how to mix the solution.

Rules for safe food preparation to prevent cholera[1]

1. Cook raw foods thoroughly

In an area affected by cholera, many raw foods, most notably fish, shellfish, and vegetables, are often contaminated with cholera bacteria. Thorough cooking will kill the bacteria, but remember that the temperature of *all parts of the food* must reach at least 70 °C. Do not eat uncooked foods, unless they can be peeled or shelled.

2. Eat cooked foods immediately

When cooked foods cool to room temperature, bacteria begin to grow. The longer the wait, the greater the risk. To be on the safe side, eat cooked foods as soon as they come off the heat. When there is a delay between cooking and eating food, as when food is sold in restaurants or by street vendors, it should be kept at 60 °C or more, over heat, until it is served.

3. Store cooked foods carefully

If you must prepare foods in advance or want to keep leftovers, be sure to store them in a refrigerator or ice-box below 10 °C or in an efficient hot-box kept continuously above 60 °C. This rule is of vital importance if you plan to store foods for more than four or five hours. Cooked foods that have been stored must be

---

[1] Adapted from Annex 6, Golden rules for safe food preparation, of *Health surveillance and management procedures for food-handling personnel: report of a WHO Consultation.* Geneva, World Health Organization, 1989 (WHO Technical Report Series, No. 785).

thoroughly reheated before eating. *Foods for infants should be eaten immediately after being prepared, and should not be stored at all.*

4. Reheat cooked foods thoroughly

Reheating foods thoroughly before eating is your best protection against bacteria that may have grown during storage. (Proper storage at low temperatures slows down the growth of bacteria but does not kill them.) Once again, thorough reheating means that *all parts of the food* must reach at least 70 °C. Eat food while it is still hot.

5. Avoid contact between raw foods and cooked foods

Safely cooked food can become contaminated through even the slightest contact with raw food. This cross-contamination can be direct, as when raw fish comes into contact with cooked foods. It can also be indirect. For example, do not prepare a raw fish and then use the same unwashed cutting surface and knife to slice cooked food. Doing so can reintroduce all the potential risks of illness that were present before cooking.

6. Choose foods processed for safety

Many foods, such as fruits and vegetables, are best in their natural state. However, in an area affected by cholera they may not be safe unless they have been processed. Canned, acidic, and dried foods should be without risk. When shopping, keep in mind that food processing was invented to improve safety as well as to prolong shelf-life.

7. Wash hands repeatedly

Wash hands thoroughly before you start preparing food and after every interruption — especially if you have to "change" or clean up the baby or have used the toilet or latrine. After preparing raw foods, such as fish or shellfish, wash your hands again before you start handling other foods.

8. Keep all kitchen surfaces clean

Since foods are so easily contaminated, any surface used for food preparation must be kept absolutely clean. Think of every food scrap, crumb or spot as a potential source of bacteria. Cloths used for washing or drying food preparation surfaces, dishes, and utensils should be changed every day and boiled before reuse. Separate cloths for cleaning the floors also require daily washing.

9. Use safe water

Safe water is just as important for food preparation as for drinking. If you have any doubts about the water supply, bring water to a rolling boil before adding it to food that will not be further cooked, or making ice for drinks. Be especially careful with any water used to prepare an infant's meal. When chlorine tablets are available, they may be used instead of boiling to make water safe.

Annex 5
Isolation of
Vibrio cholerae O1
in a peripheral laboratory

Vibrio cholerae O1, the causative agent of cholera, can be isolated and identified in any laboratory that has the basic equipment and supplies for bacteriological investigations. The vibrios are present in large numbers in the stools of patients with cholera before antibiotic therapy. They grow easily and rapidly on a variety of selective and non-selective alkaline media.

The following guidelines describe a simple and rapid method for the isolation and identification of *Vibrio cholerae* O1 in diarrhoeal stools.[1]

A5.1 Collection and transport of faecal samples

Collect the stool sample before the patient is given an antibiotic. Use a clean cotton-tipped swab, and introduce it well into the rectum. When this is done properly, the swab will become moist and may be faecally stained.

Alternatively, collect freshly passed liquid stool in a bottle or on a cotton-tipped swab.

If it is possible to be certain that the sample will reach the laboratory within 2 hours, put the rectal swab or liquid stool into a sterile screw-cap bottle; seal the bottle tightly for transport.

If, however, the specimen will not reach the laboratory within 2 hours, put it into a tube containing Cary-Blair transport medium.

---

[1] For instructions on how to isolate *Vibrio cholerae* O1 from asymptomatic carriers, and water, sewage, or food samples, see the *Manual for laboratory investigations of acute enteric infections* (Geneva, World Health Organization, 1987: unpublished WHO document CDD/83.3 Rev 1, available on request from the Programme for Control of Diarrhoeal Diseases, World Health Organization, 1211 Geneva 27, Switzerland). This manual also describes additional tests to characterize *Vibrio cholerae* O1, identify atypical isolates, and distinguish *Vibrio cholerae* O1 from other vibrios and vibrio-like organisms.

Alkaline peptone water (APW) may also be used if the transport time will not exceed 24 hours. At the laboratory, the specimen should be transferred to a fresh tube of APW for enrichment before inoculating solid media (see section A5.2).

When a transport medium is not available, soak strips of blotting paper with liquid stool. Send them to the laboratory in carefully sealed plastic bags to prevent drying.

Transport specimens in refrigerated boxes, if possible, or at ambient temperature.

A5.2 Culture and initial identification of *Vibrio cholerae* O1

Select and inoculate solid media

Laboratory technicians who are not experienced in identifying vibrios should use a selective medium and, if possible, a non-selective one. As experience is gained in recognizing typical colonies, the process may be simplified by using only the non-selective medium.

Satisfactory non-selective media include:

- meat extract agar (MEA), pH 8.5
- gelatin agar (GA), pH 8.2 to 8.5.

  Satisfactory selective media include:

- thiosulfate citrate bile salts agar (TCBS agar), pH 8.6

  Note: TCBS plates should be used within 3 days of being prepared.

- taurocholate tellurite gelatin agar (TTGA), pH 8.5.

  Instructions on preparing these media are given in section A5.3.

  If possible, both the following procedures for inoculating the medium should be followed:

(1) Streak the specimen directly onto a non-selective or selective medium, or onto both. Incubate the plates overnight (12–18 hours) at 35–37 °C.
(2) Enrich the culture of *Vibrio cholerae* O1 by inoculating the swab, or by putting 2–3 loopfuls of stool into a tube of APW. Incubate the specimen for 6–8 hours at 35–37 °C.

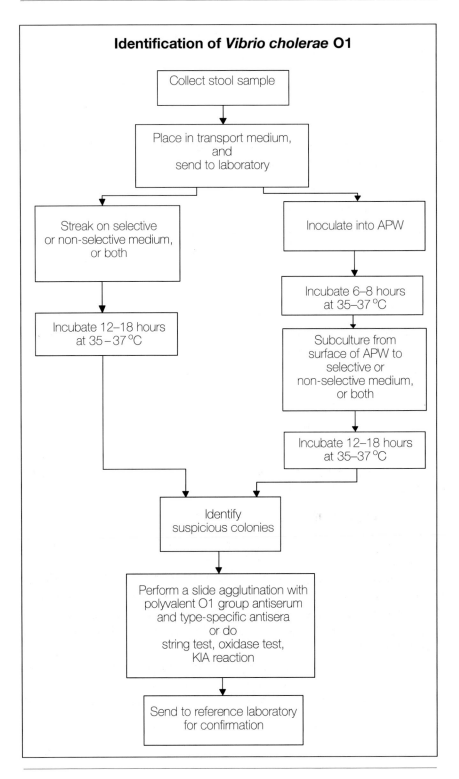

Identification of *Vibrio cholerae* O1

Collect stool sample

Place in transport medium,
and
send to laboratory

Streak on selective
or non-selective medium,
or both

Inoculate into APW

Incubate 12–18 hours
at 35–37 °C

Incubate 6–8 hours
at 35–37 °C

Subculture from
surface of APW to
selective or
non-selective medium,
or both

Incubate 12–18 hours
at 35–37 °C

Identify
suspicious colonies

Perform a slide agglutination with
polyvalent O1 group antiserum
and type-specific antisera
or do
string test, oxidase test,
KIA reaction

Send to reference laboratory
for confirmation

Then, inoculate plates from the APW tube and incubate as in (1) above.

If the incubation of APW exceeds 8 hours, inoculate a second tube of APW from the first, and repeat the incubation for 6–8 hours before inoculating solid media.

If only one procedure is followed, enrichment in APW followed by inoculation of solid media is recommended.

Identify suspicious colonies

Colonies of *Vibrio cholerae* O1 and *Vibrio cholerae* non-O1 have the same appearance:

- On MEA, they are colourless, translucent, flat, and 2–3 mm in diameter.
- On GA, they appear the same as on MEA, but have a halo.
- On TCBS agar, they are yellow, shiny, convex, and 2–3 mm in diameter. (Some strains of *Aeromonas* have a similar appearance.)
- On TTGA, they are translucent, flat, and 1–2 mm in diameter. At 24 hours they have dark pinpoint centres; later the colonies become gun-metal grey.

Perform tests to make a presumptive identification of *Vibrio cholerae* O1

Slide agglutination with specific antisera

Suspicious colonies should be tested for slide agglutination in polyvalent (group) *Vibrio cholerae* O1 antiserum.

Colonies may be tested directly from MEA, GA, or TTGA media. However, colonies from TCBS agar should not be tested directly because they are difficult to emulsify. Yellow colonies from TCBS agar should first be subcultured on MEA or GA for serological testing.

If possible, positive reactions should be confirmed with monovalent Ogawa and Inaba typing sera. *Vibrio cholerae* O1 will react with the O1 group antiserum *and* either Ogawa or Inaba typing serum.

A rapid presumptive diagnosis of *Vibrio cholerae* O1 can be attempted by streaking stool heavily on a pre-dried MEA or GA plate. This specimen should be incubated for 4–6 hours at 35 – 37 °C, and the confluent growth from the plate used to test for slide agglutination.

Other useful tests

Performing the above test with specific antisera is sufficient to diagnose a case of cholera when clinical and/or epidemiological patterns also suggest the disease.

However, if the required antisera are not available, the following tests may be used to support the identification of *Vibrio cholerae* O1, but will not differentiate serogroup O1 from other serogroups.

- *String test.* Suspend an 18- to 24-hour growth from an MEA, GA, or TTGA plate, or a Kligler's iron agar (KIA) slant in a drop of 0.5% aqueous solution of sodium desoxycholate on a slide.

  When positive, the suspension immediately loses turbidity and becomes mucoid (as with all vibrios). A mucoid "string" forms when the loop is drawn slowly away from the suspension. A few strains of *Aeromonas* show a weak string after about 60 seconds.

- *Oxidase test.* Use fresh growth from an MEA, GA, or TTGA plate, or the KIA slant (but not a TCBS agar plate). All *Vibrio cholerae* (both O1 and non-O1) are oxidase-positive, as are a number of other Gram-negative bacteria. However, Enterobacteriaceae are oxidase-negative. (See section A5.3 for further instructions.)

- *Kligler's iron agar (KIA) reaction.* Inoculate suspicious colonies into a tube of KIA. *Vibrio cholerae* (both O1 and non-O1) produce an alkaline (red) slant, acid (yellow) butt, and no hydrogen sulfide or other gas. Some other Gram-negative bacteria also produce this reaction.

Send specimen to a reference laboratory for confirmation

Laboratory diagnosis of *Vibrio cholerae* O1, as described above, can be completed within 24 – 48 hours in a peripheral laboratory, and is sufficient for most purposes. However, when additional studies are desired to confirm cholera or to identify atypical isolates, these can be done at a reference laboratory. Such studies may include serotyping, biotyping, antibiotic sensitivity testing, and biochemical characterization of suspected *Vibrio cholerae* O1. They may also involve identification of atypical strains or related species.

A nutrient agar or trypticase soy agar (TSA) stab should be used to transport the specimen to a reference laboratory.

Note: In most cases, the specimen would be sent to a national reference laboratory. Special tests and training for laboratory staff, however, can be arranged with some international reference laboratories (see section 9.2).

A5.3 Preparation of media for transporting and isolating *Vibrio cholerae* O1

Media such as Cary-Blair, TCBS agar, and KIA are best provided to laboratories as premixed dry ingredients. However, other media can be prepared at the peripheral laboratory, according to the following instructions. (For more information on the composition of various media, see *Manual for laboratory investigations of acute enteric infections*.)

Alkaline peptone water (APW)

Peptone .... 10 g
Sodium chloride .... 10 g
Distilled water .... 1000 ml

Preparation. Add ingredients to the water and adjust pH to 8.5 with a concentrated solution of sodium hydroxide. Dispense in 5–10 ml amounts into screw-capped bottles. Autoclave at 121 °C for 15 minutes. (Store alkaline media in bottles with tightly screwed caps to prevent a drop in pH.)

Meat extract agar (MEA)

Peptone .... 10 g
Sodium chloride.................... 10 g
Meat extract (concentrate)... 3 g
Agar.. 20 g
Distilled water....................... 1000 ml

Preparation. Add ingredients to the water and heat to boiling while stirring to dissolve the agar. Adjust the pH to 8.5 with a concentrated solution of sodium hydroxide. Autoclave at 121 °C for 15 minutes. Pour plates aseptically (20 ml per plate). Allow plates to cool slowly and store them in an inverted position at 4 °C. The plates should be used within 3–5 days.

Note: On this medium, colonies of *Vibrio cholerae* O1 are translucent, whereas those of Enterobacteriaceae are opaque.

Gelatin agar (GA)

Peptone	4 g
Yeast extract	1 g
Gelatin	15 g
Sodium chloride	10 g
Agar	15 g
Distilled water	1000 ml

Preparation. Add ingredients to the water and heat to boiling while stirring to dissolve the agar. Adjust pH to 8.5 with a concentrated solution of sodium hydroxide. Dispense into screw-capped bottles. Autoclave at 121 °C for 15 minutes.

Taurocholate tellurite gelatin agar (TTGA)

Trypticase	10 g
Sodium chloride	10 g
Sodium taurocholate	5 g
Sodium carbonate	1 g
Gelatin	30 g
Agar	15 g
Distilled water	1000 ml

Preparation. Add ingredients to the water and heat to boiling while stirring to dissolve the agar. Adjust the pH to 8.5 with a concentrated solution of sodium hydroxide. Dispense into screw-capped bottles. Autoclave at 121 °C for 15 minutes.

Before use, add 0.5–1.0 ml of a filter-sterilized 0.1% aqueous solution of potassium tellurite to each 100 ml of the melted TTGA medium at 55 °C. Mix well. Pour plates aseptically (20 ml per plate).

A5.4 Oxidase reagent and test

Oxidase reagent is a 1% solution of tetramethyl-*p*-phenylenediamine dihydrochloride in distilled water. (1% dimethyl-*p*-phenylenediamine may also be used in the paper strip test.)

The reagent should be colourless and should be stored in a glass-stoppered, dark brown bottle, protected from the light, in a refrigerator. If only a clear glass bottle is available, it should be wrapped in aluminium foil or dark paper.

The oxidase test is performed as follows:

Use fresh growth from an MEA, GA, or TTGA plate, or the KIA slant (but not a TCBS agar plate). Place 2–3 drops of the oxidase reagent on a piece of filter paper in a Petri dish. Smear the culture across the wet paper with a platinum (not nichrome) loop or a clean, fine wooden toothpick.

A positive reaction is indicated by the appearance of a dark purple colour on the paper within 10 seconds. Among the Gram-negative rods, *Vibrio, Campylobacter, Aeromonas, Plesiomonas, Pseudomonas,* and *Alcaligenes* are oxidase-positive. All Enterobacteriaceae are negative.

Test a positive control using a species of *Pseudomonas* and a negative control using a strain of *Escherichia coli* at the same time.